Energise

Energise

100 natural ways to feeling great

Carol Morley & Liz Wilde

MQP
MQ Publications Ltd

introduction

Are you tired all the time? Do you regularly have low-energy days when even the thought of getting out of bed makes you feel exhausted? Poor energy levels can be due to stress, diet and even boredom. Stress sends an adrenalin rush through your body that uses up precious energy needed to keep the rest of you going. The food you eat supplies your body with energy, but if you're not eating enough of the right stuff, you won't have sufficient fuel to last you through the day. And if you're stuck in a rut and bored with life, your mind (quickly followed by your body) will kick back and start working part-time. Understand what's sapping your energy levels and you can make a serious difference to your life. Just small changes will leave you re-energised and ready to go. This little book tells you how.

contents

chapter 1

Eating for energy

1 Carbohydrates are the best energy foods as they release sugar slowly into your bloodstream. For a quick fix eat wholemeal bread, rice and dried fruit like raisins and apricots. For a slow, steady burn, choose complex carbohydrates like porridge, pasta, potatoes and muesli. But steer clear of starches such as white pasta, bread and rice, as these will send you off to sleep.

2 Choose foods containing nutrients that allow your body to convert food into energy.

Vitamin B – avocado, tuna, yogurt, chicken, eggs

Vitamin C – broccoli, Brussels sprouts, citrus fruit, green peppers, tomatoes

Vitamin E – asparagus, mangoes, brazil nuts, sunflower seeds, spinach

Iron – eggs, meat, shellfish, cereal, chickpeas, dried fruit

Magnesium – spinach, broccoli, grapefruit, apples, cashew nuts

Potassium – potatoes, raisins, pistachios, sunflower seeds

Zinc – brown rice, seaweed, pumpkin seeds, cashew nuts.

11

3 **When stress is sapping your energy, counteract the attack with plenty of energy-giving foods.** Fill up on food in its natural state, such as raw fruit and vegetables, wholegrain bread, nuts and seeds.

14

4 **Eating for energy in a nutshell:**

Natural whole foods

= *energy givers*

Fatty, refined and highly processed foods

= *energy sappers*

Make every mouthful something that gives you energy, not takes it away.

5 **In-Flight Energy Foods:**

- *Dried fruit (mango, dates and figs)*
- *Nuts (almonds, pistachios, walnuts and cashews)*
- *Bananas*
- *Bottled water (have a glass every hour you're airborne).*

6 **A clove of garlic a day will help you on your way** as it contains a mineral called germanium which boosts your body's energy production.

7 **Foods most likely to fuel you are plant-based** so fill your fridge with fresh fruit and vegetables. Green leafy vegetables contain vitamins C & E, betacarotene, zinc and iron – all nutrients that energise your body and brain. Make yourself energy-packed raw juices such as carrot and beetroot to get you buzzing. Buy wholegrain bread and pasta, and brown rice. And choose the choicer cut of meat (ie lean and low-fat) or fill up on fish. Vegetarian? No problem. Let beans be your protein punch.

8 **Bouncing blood sugar plays havoc with your energy levels.** Heavy meals make you dip, so stay stable by eating three light meals a day with healthy snacks in between. For a sweet fix, snack on seedless white grapes rather than caffeine-packed chocolate.

9 **Food gives your body energy, but not before taking some away during digestion,** which is why you feel so tired after too much munching. Choose foods that break down fast – raw fruit and vegetables, nuts and seeds, brown rice, tofu and extra virgin olive oils. In second place comes wholemeal bread, chicken, fish and goat's milk. Heavyweight foods include red meat (which takes two days to digest), white bread and rice, microwaved food, sugar and cow's milk dairy products.

10 Ditch the diet. Food provides your body with energy, and the less you eat, the less you'll have. Calories are the energy we need to lead a healthy life, but the trick is to match the amount of calories you eat with the amount you burn up. Even when relaxing, your body is busy working, and if you're concentrating, all the better (the average brain uses about one calorie every four minutes). Very light work such as cooking burns between 80–100 calories an hour, moderate exercise like housework burns between 110–160 and more serious exercise such as cycling or fast walking an impressive 170–240.

11 Bananas are the ultimate feel-good food. They're rich in fibre and starch for quick-release, slow-acting energy and also contain mood-enhancing ingredients such as vitamin B6 and tryptophan. Much better than a bar of chocolate.

12 **Feeling tired may just be a sign that you're dehydrated.** Water is essential to the energy production going on in the cells of your body. Gulping two glasses of water will wake you up in minutes, and the faster you drink, the bigger energy surge you'll feel.

13 **Coffee addicts should switch to decaffeinated beans,** but beware the type of process used to make them that way. Some involve using similar solvents to those found in paint strippers and dry-cleaning solutions. The coffee is then steamed to bring the chemical level back down to legal limits, but residues can remain. Play safe by choosing coffee that's been decaffeinated using a water-only process – read the small print before buying.

14 **For a healthy hot drink high, try sipping rosehip tea** which gives you energy without the caffeine payback later. Or make your own energising ginger tea by grating a small dessertspoon of fresh ginger into your hand and squeezing into hot water.

15 **What you eat (or don't eat) for breakfast determines how much energy you'll have for the rest of the day.** A cup of coffee simply won't cut it. What you need is a real meal that includes carbohydrates, protein and fat. Eat a carbo-charged breakfast (plain toast, muffin or bagel) and your energy will last a couple of hours. Add slower-burning protein and fat to your plate and you'll be buzzing all morning. Brilliant (and tasty) breakfasts include wholegrain toast and peanut butter, poached or scrambled eggs on toast or a wholewheat bagel and smoked salmon. Or try the model's favourite, a bowl of porridge. This complex carbohydrate releases energy slowly all day, making it perfect for when you're too busy for lunch. Not a morning person? Then it's even more important to find time for a breakfast fix.

16 **The oilier the fish, the more omega-3 fatty acids it contains.** These workaholics transport oxygen, remove cholesterol, lower blood pressure and support the nervous system, all the better to cope with stress. And if this wasn't enough, fatty fish also ups energy levels by boosting your heart and circulation.

17 **Treat yourself to a Japanese meal at the end of an exhausting day.** Seaweed is known to boost energy levels, and a bowl of miso soup plus a seaweed salad will ensure you leave the restaurant with more bounce than when you went in.

18 **If you're suffering from a serious energy slump** (and you're not ill), a nutritionist will know where you're going wrong. By checking which nutrients you're lacking, an expert can prescribe an eating plan to get you back on top form.

19 **When you've overdone the eating, your body has to clear the clutter, which takes even more energy than usual.** A mini fast could be just what your body needs to give it a break. Try eating only raw fresh fruit and vegetables for a whole day after over-indulgence. Drink plenty of water to help your body with the elimination process, and be aware that the more toxins in your body, the worse you're going to feel. Take it easy and plan a relaxing day while your insides are hard at work.

20 **Seeds and grains are packed with energy-giving goodness.** Buy bags in your local supermarket and grow your own. Use chickpeas, lentils and mung beans in salads and soups, or pop in your pocket for a snack without the slump. Soak seeds overnight, line a tray with nylon mesh to encourage drainage and pour in. Place in a warm dark spot for three days, spraying twice a day with water, then transfer to a sunny spot for a few hours before eating.

chapter 2

Exercise high

21 **Exercise regularly and you'll have more energy. That's a fact.** In studies, women who'd never lifted a weight in their lives, started to keep fit and suddenly had almost 30% more energy than ever before. But what if you've not got the energy to start in the first place? Begin slowly and remember, any amount of activity makes you feel better than crashing out on the sofa.

Need more convincing? Shock statistic: Researchers say that failing to exercise can be as harmful to your health as smoking a half pack of cigarettes a day. Now that's what we call an incentive.

22 **Heard of a runner's high?** Well, it's true. After a heart-pumping run, you'll feel you can take on the world. That's because exercise stimulates the body's pituitary gland which releases those feel-good endorphins. Research shows it's almost impossible to feel bad about yourself after a workout. Just don't sign up for that marathon until you've come down to earth.

23 Whatever you're doing, if you're fit you'll be able to do it better. That means dancing, gardening, sex and even shopping, because exercise improves your stamina. They'll have to drag you off the dance floor.

24 Modern fitness no longer means gruelling hours spent at the gym. Just thirty minutes, three times a week of any activity that gets your body breathing harder than normal will up your energy levels, relieve depression, oh, and give you the body you've always dreamed of.

25 **Walking is the best energy fix around.** It not only increases your intake of oxygen and boosts your immune system, but also stimulates a tired body and mind. Walk briskly for at least 30 minutes, or make that an hour and you'll be happy to know you've also burnt off around 400 calories.

26 **Always feel lethargic after lunch?** Then head out for a 10 minute walk. Studies show this boosts energy for up to two hours after your stroll.

27 **Nowadays it's easier to send an e-mail than walk to another office for a chat.** We all know we should be active, but fewer than half of us are. So tear yourself away from your screen once in a while and go visit your friend on the 5th floor. If your boss catches you, blame it on a computer break – you're legally entitled.

28 **Another link between energy and exercise.** You can't feel energetic without the right foods to fuel you, and regular activity improves your body's ability to break down food by upping the oxygen levels in your bloodstream and increasing the efficiency of your heart.

29 **Weight training's not just for meat-heads.** A stronger body equals more energy. Why? The weaker you are, the more energy you need to keep going. So build more muscle and life will be a breeze.

30 **When you've been ill, your body needs to rest and repair.** But vegging out in the house for days and days will leave you weak and even more vulnerable to illness. Once you're on the mend, the longer you stay on your sick bed (or sofa), the more tired you'll feel. But beware sudden activity which will leave you exhausted. Take it gently. Any new exercise routine needs to be done for at least a week before your muscles get used to the shock and you can crank up the pace.

31 **Even a gentle stretch can improve your energy levels and also helps calm a stressed-out mind.** Stretching expands your chest area, giving your inner organs more room to operate. The result? Increased blood flow and more energy-giving oxygen rushing around inside you. Just a few minutes a day will do the job.

1. Stand up straight with your feet hip width apart and your fingers interlocked behind your head.

2. Take a deep breath in and as you breathe out, push your arms up with palms facing upwards. At the same time, feel your whole body stretching towards the ceiling.

3. Relax down and repeat until you feel loose and lengthened.

41

32 **Exercising in the fresh air clears your head and inspires your mind.** Cycling in the great outdoors is far more interesting than watching a row of gym-bound bikers, and outdoor exercise works you harder too. Consider the difference between a stationary bike in the gym and the open road. You're guaranteed to burn more calories as you power your bike up hills, round corners and into the wind. Far more energetic than reading a magazine propped up on the handlebars as you pedal.

33 **You're never going to feel full of beans if you're feeling blue,** but studies prove that regular exercise beats depression. Just four weeks of activity can seriously improve your mood. Guaranteed.

34 **You know regular exercise makes you feel better,** but you keep pushing that snooze button in the mornings until it's too late for anything more than a shower. It's hard to keep yourself motivated when exercising alone, but become part of a team and you'll find it tough to say no.

Choose something you fancy – basketball, football, tennis, a running club – and let your fellow exercisers inspire you. And don't worry if they're all so much more skilled than you. Do what you can and you'll soon catch up with the rest of them.

35 **OK, so exercise can give you energy, but heading for the gym straight after a long tiring day will just make you feel worse.** Instead, go home and get a good night's sleep and save your exercising for the next morning. And remember, vigorous exercise too late at night will stimulate your mind and body, making it harder to fall asleep later.

36 **Don't be tempted to spend Saturday making up for your lack of exercise all week.** A sudden burst of activity will leave you feeling exhausted, not energised. Instead, work exercise into the week, even if you're only walking to the bus stop and back. As with most things, little and often is better than all or nothing.

37 **Ancient martial arts are the very latest way to get fit.** Expect gentle movements in t'ai chi and qigong, where the emphasis is on internal strength and a calmer mind. More physical by far are karate and judo – you'll learn a serious method of self-defence while getting a great workout. Whatever you choose, all martial arts aim to energise the mind and body, sharpen reflexes, improve coordination and promote mental relaxation.

38 **Exercise doesn't just give your body energy – it energises your mind too.** Research has found that regular activity three times a week improves memory and judgement by 25%.

can try anything from power yoga, pilates, kickboxing, spinning to boot camp (pretend you're in the army). First timers should look for classes with the magic words 'beginner' or 'basic' in the title, and

39 **Are you allergic to aerobics?** Gym classes have come a long way since leg-warmer-wearing instructors high-kicked along to 1980s disco tunes. Now you

48

go along with a friend if you're shy. Just remember to keep your eye on the teacher and if you lose the plot, march on the spot rather than stop dead in your tracks. Like any skill, expect to take

40 **For the maximum heart-pumping, fat-burning high, vary the intensity of your work-out** (known in the trade as interval training). A heart that goes up and down is working far harder than one that stays on the same level.

a few lessons to learn the ropes, and for the ultimate energy high, pick an instructor who shares your taste in music. After 30 minutes of feel-good tunes, you'll be flying.

chapter 3

Energy enemies

41 **Couch-potato pursuits such as watching TV will leave you more tired then ever.** Lying in front of the box all night is never going to fill you with energy. Think about it. When was the last time you switched off the TV and jumped up ready for anything? Chances are, by the end of the night you've hardly got the energy to hunt for the remote control.

42 **Work, home, bills, shopping, family commitments. No wonder adults don't have nearly as much energy as children.** You may not be able to avoid the responsibilities of being a grown-up, but you can still find time to play like a child. Taking life too seriously will definitely sap your energy.

43 **Coffee and other caffeinated drinks (think hot chocolate, cola and tea), give you an instant high, quickly followed by a low,** made much worse if you were tired in the first place. Drinking coffee to boost your energy will just set you off on a downward spiral, so stick to three cups a day max and for every one you down, drink twice as much water to make up for it (caffeine is also a diuretic). Or switch to tea, which gives a more subtle roller-coaster ride.

44 **Sugar works in the same way, shooting straight into your bloodstream.** The result? Your blood sugar level rises too rapidly, making your body race to lower it again. Expect an energy slump between one and three hours after tucking into a sugary snack.

45 **A walk by the seaside or a ramble in the country leaves you buzzing with energy. Why?** Because fresh air is charged with negative ions, which stimulate the oxygenation of the blood and energise your body. No surprises then, that you feel your lowest surrounded by car fumes, electrical equipment, synthetic materials (ie carpets, curtains and a cheaply covered sofa), cigarette smoke and air conditioning, which all reduce the level of negative ions. Another excuse to escape somewhere green at the weekend.

46 **Step out the front door and your body is bombarded with toxins.** These all put pressure on your immune system to work overtime, resulting in less energy for the rest of you. Do yourself a favour and don't add to the toxic overload by smoking. Inhaling cigarette smoke (and even passive smoking) exposes you to over 200 chemicals each time you (or someone else) lights up. And smoking also deprives your body of energy-giving oxygen and constricts your blood vessels, slowing circulation and making your heart work twice as fast to compensate. Give up now and experience an energy boost almost immediately.

47 **When stress levels are sky-high, your body suffers an adrenalin rush,** which releases fatty acids and glucose into the bloodstream. As these are your body's main energy supply, a change in circulation will leave you low. Some stress is good for motivation, but severe stress can carry a serious health warning. Much of stress is within your control. Decipher what (or who) drives you mad and fathom how to cut it (or them) out of your life.

48 **Boredom drains your energy far more than being busy doing things you enjoy.** If you're stuck in a rut, climb out. A lack of new challenges will leave you lazy and apathetic.

49 **aMany of us spend the day under outdated fluorescent strip lighting** which was only designed to be a cheap, short-term way to extend working hours in times of darkness. Scientists have discovered that people who spend most of their time away from natural light suffer fatigue, headaches and depression. Swap your lighting to full-spectrum bulbs (which simulate natural daylight), or get outside as often as you can for an instant lift. Artificial light actually suppresses the production of a hormone found in humans called melatonin. The same hormone in animals is responsible for hibernation patterns, so no wonder a day under strip lighting leaves you feeling lethargic.

62

50 When you're tired and low, you may feel the only way to get through the evening is with a glass of wine permanently in your hand. But alcohol is a depressant. Sure, it may not feel like that at first, but wait until the alcohol hits your brain (about 20% gets there in seconds). It slows down both your movement and your mind. Not to mention the morning after come-down. No one feels full of energy with a hangover.

51 One or two glasses of wine can calm you down after a bad day, but any more will stop you sleeping soundly, making you feel even more miserable the next morning.

52 Negative people bring you down. Surround yourself with miserable people, and it won't be long before you're moaning too. And that goes for bad relationships. They're a waste of time and energy, so get out now. Stuck with a rude, ungrateful boss? Find someone else who appreciates your skills.

53 Don't underestimate the power of your mind. If you've suffered a traumatic event, your mind will need extra energy to cope, which leaves your body in short supply. So be kind to yourself and take life easy until you're over the worst.

54 Candida is a yeast-like fungus which goes into overdrive when your body's good bacteria is attacked (the contraceptive pill and antibiotics can do the damage). Symptoms include thrush, IBS, bloating, constipation and diarrhoea, and serious fatigue. If your energy levels are low, you'll need an anti-fungal product to fight off the fungus, and a low-yeast, low-sugar diet will also help as fungus feeds on these foods. Cut out all sugar and alcohol, eat only fresh fruit in the morning. Resist bread, pasta and pizza, and ditch the dairy (eat soya and goat's milk products instead).

55 **It's not only sleep you're missing when you spend your nights in dark discos and bars.** It's fresh air too. Add the two together and guess who's going to feel flat the next day?

56 **Feeling under the weather is your body's warning sign** that you've got an energy crisis on your hands. Listen and learn from it.

57 **If you regularly suffer nodding head syndrome mid afternoon,** chances are you're stuck in a centrally heated room. Any atmosphere with a low humidity level will make you feel tired and lethargic, and most double-glazed offices are way too low. Place bowls of water around radiators or invest in a humidifier to beat the post-lunch slump.

67

58 Sore shoulders? Stiff neck?

Muscular problems use up large amounts of energy, leaving little for the rest of your body to make it through the day. Take a break, stretch, treat yourself to a massage, visit an osteopath. Whatever it takes to sort out your aches and pains. Your body will thank you for it.

59 If you suffer recurring digestive problems

(think irritable bowel syndrome and bloating), low energy levels even after a good night's sleep, regular headaches and even migraine attacks, chances are you may be sensitive to something you're putting in your mouth. While serious food allergies are downright dangerous, many more minor problems can be caused by a food intolerance. Migraine sufferers are often sensitive to cheese, chocolate, citrus fruit and wine, while wheat can cause bloating and dairy products a blocked-up nose. To make matters more complicated, the very food that could be causing your problem may be the one you crave. Try cutting down on potentially unfriendly foods one at a time, or visit a dietician who'll be able to spot a food link much faster.

60 **Negative thoughts drain your energy.** Instead of thinking the worst, or mulling over potential problems, visualise yourself in a positive setting and you gain energy from it. Don't think about going on holiday with all the complicated arrangements – imagine yourself already there. Visualise new opportunities such as a dream job, a new house or a different environment. Your subconscious mind will respond to positive thoughts and act on them.

chapter 4

Energy friends

61 Natural light is an essential nutrient for your immune system. Make sure you spend some time outside every day and ditch the wraparound sunglasses occasionally when it's not too bright so you get your full sunlight fix. Light therapy doesn't only work to cure the symptoms of SAD. Putting different-coloured bulbs around your house can affect your energy levels too. If you want to feel full of vitality, sit under a bright orangey-red light. Both yellow and pink light has a feel-good factor, and blue bulbs will help you calm down at the end of a stressful day.

62 Twenty-first century technology can seriously sap your energy. Surround yourself with green plants both at home and in the office to help break down radiation coming from computers and televisions. The extra oxygen plants produce is an added energy saver.

63 Doing something daring will give you an instant energy boost. Excite your senses by swimming in a dark or floodlit pool. Make that a skinny dip for a guaranteed daredevil experience.

64 Response to sound is one of our earliest senses and research has found that a new-born baby can recognise a piece of music played before they were even born. Music has been used in healing for thousands of years to energise and help express feelings, and we instinctively use music to heal at home by choosing what makes us feel good. Avoid listening to continuous background music and instead be aware of your emotional response to different songs. When you're tired or down, play upbeat music that makes you want to dance or something that brings back memories of happier times.

65 Find your energy hot spot with a little DIY acupressure. Locate the point between your thumb and forefinger and pinch it firmly with your other hand. Hold for a minute or two and gradually release.

66 **Start your mornings on the right note.** Switch your radio alarm to a soothing station for a gentle wake up call. There's nothing worse for your mood than being woken by loud bells and buzzers.

67 **Make time to have a good time.** Ever wondered why children are always so full of beans? They're enjoying life.

68 **Energy-giving breath** = slow and deep from the abdomen. **Energy-sapping breath** = quick and shallow from the chest. **The best breath** = as you breathe in, your lungs expand to push out your tummy, and as you breathe out your tummy contracts to push out air. Lie on the floor and place one hand on your stomach to feel the movement. Consciously push out your stomach as you breathe in and pull in as you breathe out. Your body will naturally follow this pattern on the next breath. Keep it up for a few minutes until you become familiar with the feeling.

69 **Feel your body fading?** Give yourself a quick foot massage to stimulate all your pressure points. Kick off your shoes, wiggle your toes and rotate your ankles. Then starting at your heel, massage the whole area of your foot in small circular movements. Bliss.

70 **Strange, but true. Massaging your ears will make you feel more energetic.** Begin at the earlobes and use your finger and thumb to massage all the way up to the top. An instant mood improver – honest.

79

71 **Most of us need between seven and nine hours' sleep to wake feeling refreshed,** but research says most of us don't manage it. Apart from permanent tiredness, the result of too little sleep is headaches, bad moods, poor memory and fuzzy eyes. Here are some ways of getting a better night's sleep:

• *Avoid napping through the day, even if your eyes are closing and your head is nodding.*

• *Don't exercise after 9pm, as working out increases energy levels for several hours afterwards.*

• *Don't go to bed until you feel tired. Tossing and turning is stressful,* not soothing. If you're not asleep after an hour, get up and read. You want your bed to be associated with rest, not frustration.

• *Take a warm bath 30 minutes before bedtime and add a sleepy essential oil like lavender, camomile or sandalwood, mixed in well while the water is running.*

• *Ditch the nighttime cup of cocoa. A cup of relaxing herbal tea will soothe you off to sleep far better than a caffeine-laden cup. Try special nighttime infusions or camomile tea.*

• *Warm milk has been proven to aid sleep as the protein is similar to one in the brain that regulates your body's sleep mechanism.*

82

72 Erratic living will sap your energy. Try to keep your natural body clock consistent by going to bed and getting up at roughly the same time every day. Confusing your body's rhythms confuses your mind.

73 Get going in the morning with the help of a stimulating citrus oil in your shower or bath. A few drops of lemon or grapefruit will do the trick. Drop into your bath water, drip onto your shower floor or add to a sponge and rub it all over, breathing deeply as you lather.

74 **Become open to new experiences.** Feel the fear, and enjoy it. Always fancied learning to water-ski? Wanted to act since the school pantomime? New challenges leave your body and mind buzzing. So much better than yet another night spent in front of the TV.

75 **When you're feeling tired, add a few drops of peppermint oil to a tissue and inhale frequently.** Or drip onto a cotton handkerchief and lay it over the top of your computer or a low-heat radiator. The aroma will fill your room and keep you alert throughout the day. Another way to scent your room is by dripping a little oil onto a light bulb. Turn on and the heat will do the rest. If you need to concentrate for long periods, inhale rosemary oil as you work and it'll keep your mind focused.

76 **The law of karma states that what you give, you receive back in even larger quantities.** So take time to give the gift of energy and happiness to others and they'll be only too pleased to return the favour.

77 **Low energy may mean an iron deficiency** as iron helps red blood cells bring oxygen to the brain and muscles. Find it in meats, eggs, fish, cherries, green leafy vegetables and dried fruit, or pop a pill to perk you up.

78 **Keep a mineral water spray in your bag or on your desk** and spritz your face when you're feeling bored or tired. A sure-fire way to wake up.

79 **Feng Shui practitioners say that cluttering up your home blocks the energy flow in your environment.** Even if you don't believe that a good clear-out can redirect and realign energy, there's no denying that moving around a tidy house is much less exhausting than fighting your way through a mess every morning.

80 **Ever wondered why buses are red and fast food burger bars are painted red, orange and yellow?** Colour is used every day to keep you moving and speed you up (so vacating your seat for someone else), and you can use colour yourself to supply a shot of much-needed energy.

- *When you need a boost, focus on something red, yellow or orange for a few minutes, so your mind can soak up the signals.*
- *If you're bored at work, surround yourself with orange to help bring you to life. Too much red interferes with decision-making, and too much yellow affects concentration.*
- *Buy candles in a wide range of colours, and light the one that suits your mood. Orange lifts your spirits, pink wakes you up and red sparks passion.*
- *The dull colours worn in winter can add to the depression of long, dark days, but switch to a bright colour and feel your energy levels lift immediately. If you're tired in the morning, wear something red.*

91

chapter 5

Energy treats

81 Peppermint oil is a great pick-me-up. Add six drops of oil to a large bowl of warm water and soak your feet for ten minutes.

82 Manipulate your own meridians for a DIY energy boost. Feel around the bottom of your foot, just under the pad that runs below your big toe and the start of your other toes. You should feel a 'W' shape and you need to press deeply into the middle of it. The trick is to press with your thumb as you slowly breathe out, and then repeat for three to ten minutes to really feel the benefit, before repeating on the other foot.

83 Everyone knows a long luxurious bath leaves you lethargic. Well, not necessarily. Too-hot water increases your pulse rate which drains your body, but make the water around 35 degrees and you'll climb out raring to go.

84 **For more hands-on healing at home, try a DIY Shiatsu head massage to clear your mind.**

1. Using your fingertips, work from the front of your scalp to the back of your head, using small circular movements.

2. Place one hand at the front of your head and one at the back and, moving them at the same time, work your fingers through your hair towards the top of your head, using circular movements.

3. From the base of your neck, work up to the top of your head, using circular movements. Apply firmer pressure to loosen tension.

85 **There's nothing like a massage to boost energy levels.** Most types of massage come from the East (even so-called Swedish massage) and are based on the idea of flowing energy. This built-up energy needs to be unblocked so your body can rebalance itself. The intimate contact also wakes up reflexes and feelings which activate your central nervous system. This floods your body with beneficial chemicals, boosting the immune system and promoting a feeling of deep relaxation. Add to that the release of muscle tension, and a massage is a must-have treat. Go as often as you can afford, or buy a book and learn to massage with a friend.

86 **Cold water will wake you up in the morning when you just feel like going back to bed.** If you're brave, a cold shower does the trick. Grit your teeth and turn the water to freezing for 30 seconds. Or give your body a boost before a busy evening by dipping your feet in cold water for 30 seconds at a time. Nodding off on a night out? Try holding an ice cube against your pulse points at the wrist, below your ears or behind your knees for 10 seconds.

87 **Ginseng has been used by the Chinese for years to boost energy.** This multi-talented herb works by stimulating the circulation, easing tension and increasing stamina (ginseng is popular for treating a low libido). And ginseng can also help you cope with mental and physical stress as it stimulates the release of energy-giving adrenalin into the bloodstream. Available in capsules or look for herbal teas and energy drinks containing ginseng for a mid-day boost.

ice → ← ice

88
Studies show that filling your surroundings with scent can improve your mental stamina and concentration. Choose one of these energising essential oils:

- *Black Pepper – makes you more alert*
- *Ginger – fights fatigue*
- *Bergamot – improves mood*
- *Lemon – keeps you focused and relaxed*
- *Eucalyptus – lifts depression*
- *Cinnamon – wakes up a tired mind*
- *Orange – helps concentration*
- *Ylang Ylang – works as an aphrodisiac.*

89 **Ancient Oriental medicine believes your energy (known as *chi*) flows along your meridians (think pathways) inside your body.** When these paths are blocked, your energy cannot flow freely. Treatments aim to stimulate the flow of energy by removing the blocks, and you can expect to finish one feeling full of energy yet pleasantly relaxed. Here's what's on offer:

Shiatsu (Japanese massage) – you lie on a mat while the practitioner applies pressure to particular points on your meridians with their thumbs, fingers, palms and sometimes even their elbows, knees and feet.

Reflexology – points on the hands and feet that correspond with internal organs are stimulated with the fingers and thumbs.

Acupuncture – very fine needles are applied to stimulate specific points.

Acupressure – similar to shiatsu, but only the fingers and thumbs are used.

90 **Zero balancing was developed by acupuncturist and osteopath Dr Fritz Smith in the 1970s** and aims to soothe and balance your physical and mental energies. The idea is that trauma can affect our subtle energy circulation, and zero balancing helps ease the flow. A practitioner will manipulate your whole body, moving and stretching bone-deep, which may also release emotional stress.

91 **Fans of flotation describe it as the deepest rest they've ever known.** The feeling of total weightlessness frees the brain and body from gravity, which releases vast amounts of energy and brain power. In a flotation tank, there's also no outside distraction so you can relax deeply and focus on your body. In fact, one hour of floating is said to have the restorative effects of four hours sleep, so it's not surprising you emerge with more energy.

92 **The Amazonian Indians got their kicks from guarana,** a mild stimulant containing caffeine, theophylline and tannin (all found in a cup of tea). One gram contains slightly less caffeine than a weak cuppa, and converts say it gives a much longer and better buzz. Chew guarana gum when you need to pep up your performance. Other natural energisers include aloe vera juice, kelp and coenzyme Q10, which all boost your body in a healthy way.

93 **A glass of wheatgrass juice works as a shot of energy,** especially if you drink it straight from the blender so the active ingredients can shoot straight into your bloodstream. Find wheatgrass at juice bars and health food shops everywhere.

94 **Poor diet can block your body with toxic waste,** draining toxins into the bloodstream. Fans of colonic irrigation believe that flushing your colon with many litres of water will dislodge the debris. This may not sound much of a treat, but devotees report a serious energy boost afterwards.

95 **Falling asleep when you should be concentrating?** Nip to the bathroom and splash your face with cool water. Just make sure you're wearing waterproof mascara!

96 **Your body's not the only thing that gets tired.** Your mind needs a rest too. Just as muscles repair and strengthen when you take a break from exercise, so your mind can relax and return refreshed to work. Get to know your own attention span and then take a guilt-free break to do something no more mentally taxing then filing your nails. Developing your own personal work style will get the most out of your mind.

97 **A skin scrub in the bath or shower will boost blood circulation and energise your whole body.** Fill a small muslin bag with oatmeal and a sprig of rosemary and gently rub your body all over, starting from the feet and working up.

98 **Get going with ginger.** Grate a small handful and squeeze the liquid into a bowl of hot water. Then dip a small hand towel into the mixture, wring out and hold over your lower back. This energy boosting compress also improves circulation and soothes a sore back (a common energy sapper).

99 Meditation slows down your body and mind so they can recharge their batteries. When you meditate, your heart rate decreases, your blood pressure falls and your breathing becomes much slower. Just twenty minutes of meditation adds up to a mini shut down which fans say is worth an hour's sleep. No wonder you feel so energised at the end. Try this DIY technique. Choose a quiet spot where you won't be interrupted and turn down the lights or close the curtains. Sit comfortably and imagine each part of your body relaxing, starting with your scalp and working down to your toes. Now concentrate on one neutral thought, such as a colour, and focus on deep breathing. Whenever a thought breaks through the calm, just let it go. After 20 minutes, slowly open your eyes and sit quietly for a short while before getting up.

100 Under pressure? Try this quick relaxation technique. You'll feel instantly calmer and have more energy to sort out what's worrying you: Take a deep breathe in and tense up all your muscles. Hold for 10 seconds and then release on a big breath out. Repeat a few times, breathing normally in between until you feel stronger and more able to cope.

Illustrator's dedication:
To my family

Author's dedication:
To my mother and father, and to Ben

Published by MQ Publications Limited
12 The Ivories, 6–8 Northampton Street, London, N1 2HY
Tel: 020 7359 2244 / Fax: 020 7359 1616
email: mqpublications.com

Text © Liz Wilde 2001
Illustrations © Carol Morley 2001
Interior design: Philippa Jarvis
Series Editor: Kate John

ISBN: 1-84072-033-6

3 5 7 9 0 8 6 4 2

Printed in China